G000155280

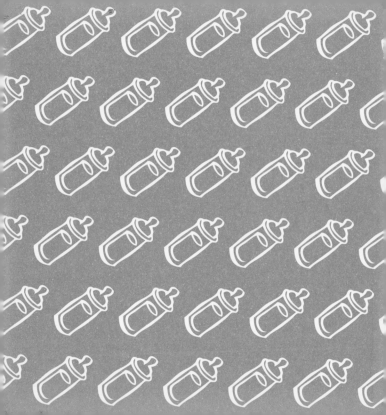

Baby Tips

help.

for
Mums

Simon Brett

summersdale

Illustrations by
Alex Hallatt

BABY TIPS FOR MUMS

This edition published 2012

First published 2005
Reprinted 2005, 2006 and 2007

Copyright © Simon Brett, 2005

Illustrations by Alex Hallatt

Summersdale Publishers Ltd
46 West Street
Chichester
West Sussex
PO19 1RP
UK

www.summersdale.com

Printed and bound in China

ISBN: 978-1-84953-282-2

Substantial discounts on bulk quantities of Summersdale books are available to corporations, professional associations and other organisations. For details telephone Summersdale Publishers on (+44-1243-771107), fax (+44-1243-786300) or email (nicky@summersdale.com).

To...

From...

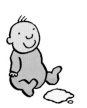

Contents

Introduction

Well, there you are. You've put in all that hard work. You've spent nine months producing what is undoubtedly the most beautiful and intelligent baby in the world, and you'd have thought the one thing you really deserve now is a nice long rest. The trouble is, that's not the way the baby sees things. Nor frequently is it the way your partner or other family members will see things. So, to help you survive what is going to be an unfairly busy stage of your life, here are a few tips...

Mum's the Word

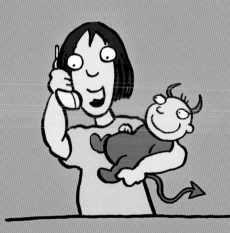

Basic Rules:

In the early weeks a new mum must prepare herself for a lot of screaming and tantrums — and that's just from her partner.

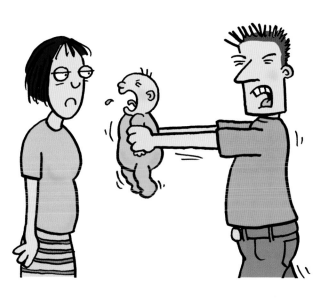

The relationship between a new mum and her baby is a power struggle... and you may as well face the fact straight away – the baby's going to win.

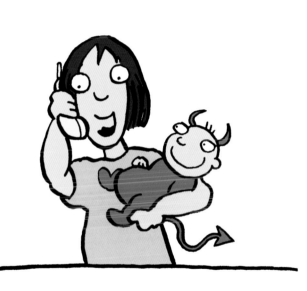

When breastfeeding,
don't think of yourself
as a canteen. Thinking
of yourself as a gourmet
restaurant is much better
for your self-esteem.

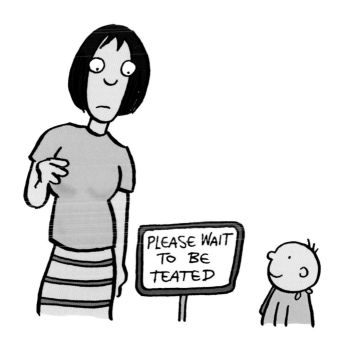

With babies, everything ends in tears... from one or other of you.

Getting your figure back
after you've had your baby
is an admirable ambition,
but then so is world
peace... and finding an NHS
dentist... and pigs flying...

When a baby is being dressed, either it seems to develop one more limb or the garment seems to develop one less hole.

The night after you said
your baby slept through the
night for the first time,
it won't.

For the convenience of
parents, baby buggies fold.
For the inconvenience of
parents, babies don't.

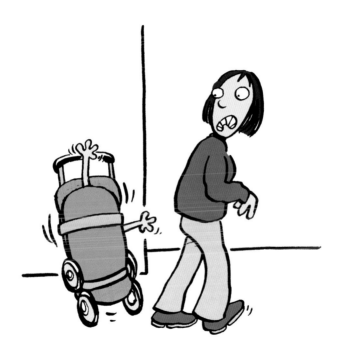

You must never say that your baby is prettier/better-natured/more intelligent than anyone else's... even though it's obviously true.

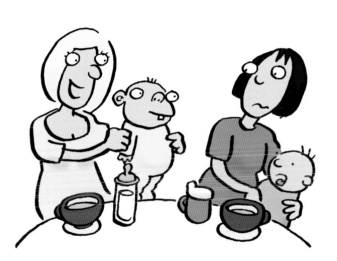

However much you would like it to be, a baby will never be a matching accessory.

You can always recognise
a new mum by:

The deep hollows under
her eyes.

You can always recognise a new mum by:

The encrustation of puke
over her shoulder.

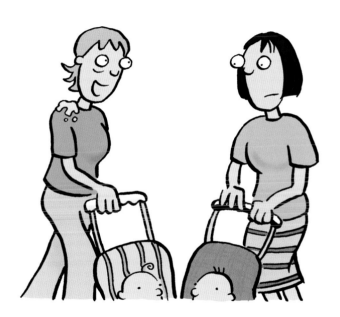

You can always recognise a new mum by:

The fact that she's still
in her dressing gown
at lunchtime.

You can always recognise a new mum by:

The lingering aroma of
sterilising fluid.

You can always recognise a new mum by:

Her inability to sustain
adult conversation.

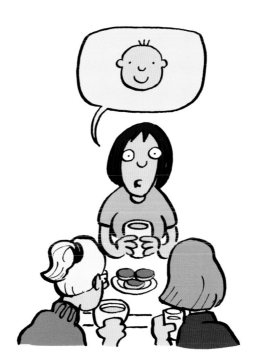

You can always recognise a new mum by:

The disappointed, neglected
look in her partner's eyes.

Daddy
Dearest

You can tell your partner
will be a good dad when:

He offers to look after the
baby while you go off for
a girlie weekend with your
friends. (Oh yes?)

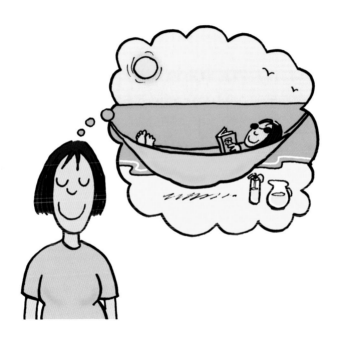

You can tell your partner will
be a good dad when:

He says, 'The baby was
crying in the night, but
you looked so peacefully
asleep that I sorted
everything out.'
(Come on!)

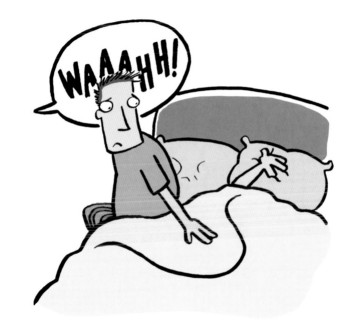

He's decided that, now he's got the responsibility of a baby, he's going to give up drinking with the boys and stay at home every evening. (Let's get back to the real world, shall we?)

Your partner should be
discouraged from:

Getting into discussions
with your mother about
A) Childcare
B) Education
C) Anything, really...

Your partner should be
discouraged from:

Wanting to dress your baby
in any team strip.

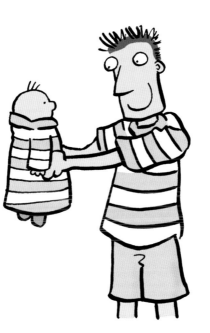

Your partner should be
discouraged from:

Asking if he can take his
paternity leave in cash and
keep working.

Your partner should be
discouraged from:

Pretending, when
you're breast-feeding in
public, that he's with
someone else.

Your partner should be
discouraged from:

Thinking that 'wetting
the baby's head' should
continue on a nightly
basis until after it's
finished school.

Mummy
Training

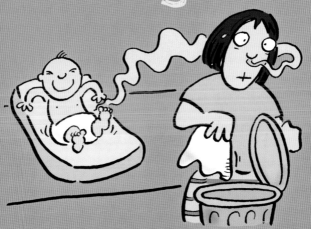

For a baby it's a point
of honour to:

Come up with an illness
which doesn't match any
of the descriptions in the
childcare books.

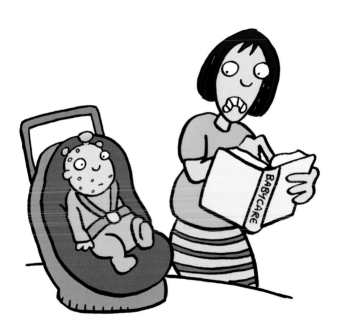

For a baby it's a point of honour to:

Hold back a really big poo
until immediately after a
nappy change.

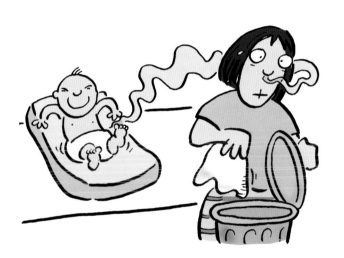

For a baby it's a point of honour to:

Listen out for the words, 'I think the baby's settled for the night now', and prove them wrong.

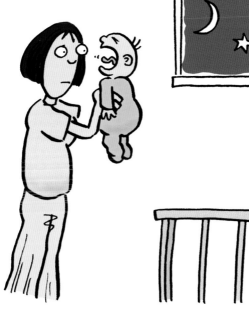

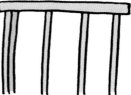

Know when its mum really wants to show it off and develop a nasty facial rash just before the event.

Be prepared for your mother
to say the following:

'You think your labour was
tough, but let me tell you,
when I had you...'

Be prepared for your mother
to say the following:

'I love your baby very
much, but I don't want to
be thought of as a free
babysitting service.'

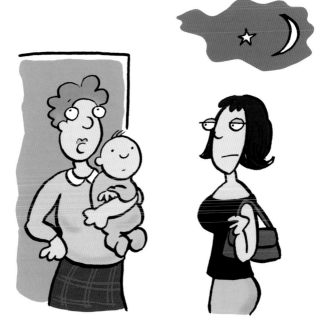

Be prepared for your mother
to say the following:

'Just because you've had a
baby, that's no excuse to
let yourself go.'

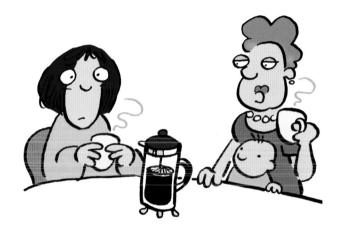

Be prepared for your mother
to say the following:

'Everybody says I look
far too young to be
a grandmother.'

The New Mum's Dictionary

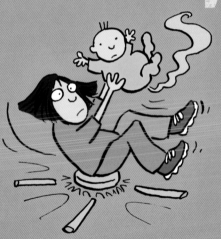

ANAEMIA: This fashion for giving babies Victorian names is really getting out of hand.

AU PAIR: A young woman whose presence in the house gives you time to yourself, and your partner ideas.

BABYSITTING CIRCLE: A reciprocal arrangement whereby parents seem to spend every night looking after other people's children and then find nobody's free on the one evening *they* want to go out.

BABY WALKER: A father at 3 a.m., having been told that 'a few turns round the block may make the baby settle'.

The New Mum's Dictionary:

BATH TIME: A daily contest between baby and parent to see who can get wetter, invariably – though unwillingly – won by the parent.

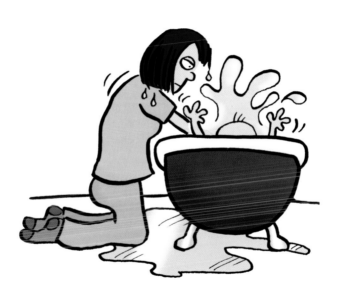

BEDTIME STORY: A childish fantasy — like, for instance, the idea that your baby goes to bed and to sleep at the same time every night.

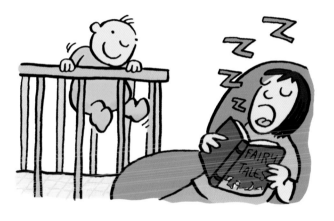

BREAST PADS: Equipment
used by women cricketers.

BURPING: Something you have to do for your baby, but which your partner can manage without any help from anyone.

The New Mum's Dictionary:

COMFORTER: Whatever works for you (partner, lover, Celine Dion CD, big box of chocolates, Maeve Binchy novel, Chardonnay, gin, etc.)

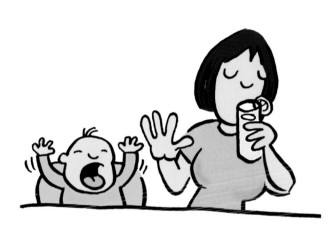

CONTRACEPTION, MOST
EFFECTIVE METHOD AFTER
BABY'S BIRTH: The baby.

FEEDING TRAY: An attachment to a high chair, something for a baby to push food off.

The New Mum's Dictionary:

HEARING TEST: The moment at the doctor's when your baby, who up until that point has been woken by the sound of a fly landing on a cushion in another room, is suddenly unable to hear a drum being banged next to its ear.

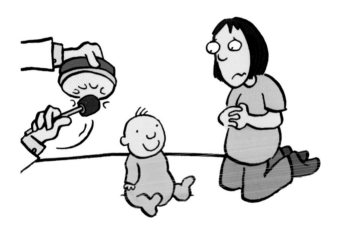

INTRODUCTION OF SOLIDS: The baby's discovery that Lego bricks fit into its mouth.

LABOUR: The process of giving birth, so called because it's BLOODY HARD WORK.

LOOSE STOOLS: The curse of
IKEA strikes again.

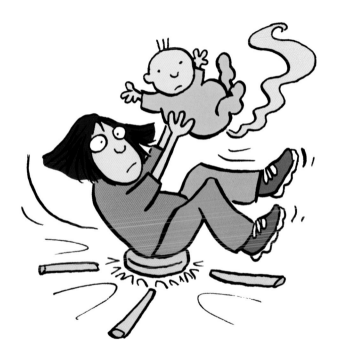

NAPPY RASH: All-purpose explanation for any bad behaviour from baby.

OTHER MUMS: Most probably, your salvation. There'll always be one who's worse at the whole business than you are.

PARENTAL DISCIPLINE: When there's a new baby in the house, it is important to establish who's boss. But don't worry about it. Most parents come into line pretty quickly.

PROJECTILE VOMITING:
Shooting from the lip.

ROLE MODEL: Someone who has completely got her figure back after having a baby.

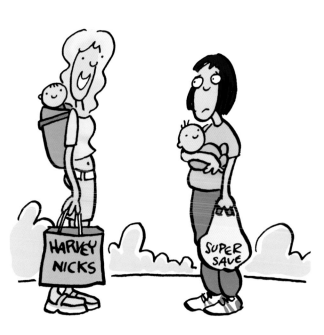

ROLL MODEL: A) What you look like, having completely failed to get your figure back after having a baby.
B) The little figurine of a ROLE MODEL you make out of bread, to stick pins in.

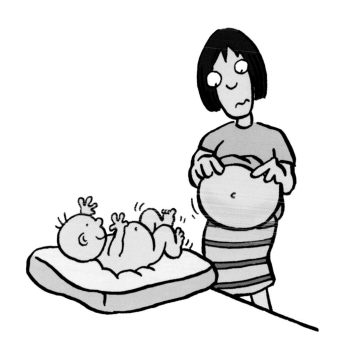

STERILISATION: Procedure recommended for dirty nappies and dirty-minded partners.

TEETHING: All-purpose explanation for any bad behaviour from baby.

The New Mum's Dictionary:

TEETHING RING: A group of babies who all decide to whinge at the same time.

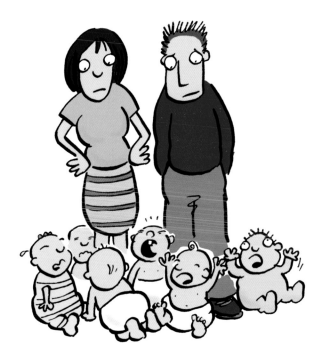

WEANING: Getting your baby off the breast. Any baby worth its salt can make this process last for years.

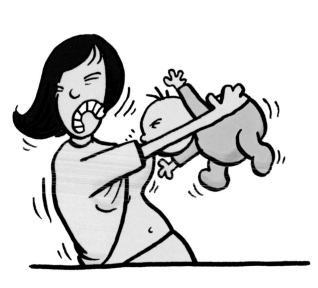

The New Mum's Dictionary:

WIND: All-purpose
explanation for any bad
behaviour from baby.

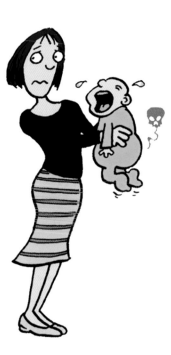

A final thought...

When your baby's being a right little pain, and you see a sign reading 'Baby Changing Facilities'... don't even think about it.

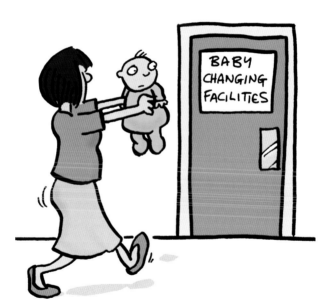

BABY
CHANGING
FACILITIES

If you're interested in finding out more
about our humour books follow us
on Twitter: @SummersdaleLOL

www.summersdale.com

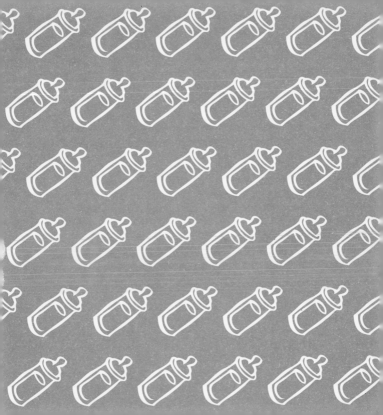

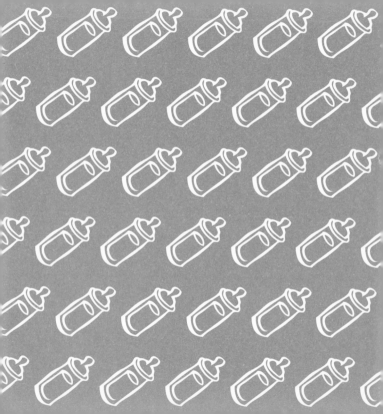